Medical Terminology

45 Mins or Less to EASILY Breakdown the Language of Medicine NOW!

Chase Hassen
Nurse Superhero

Disclaimer:

TABLE OF CONTENTS

First, I want to give you this FREE gift...

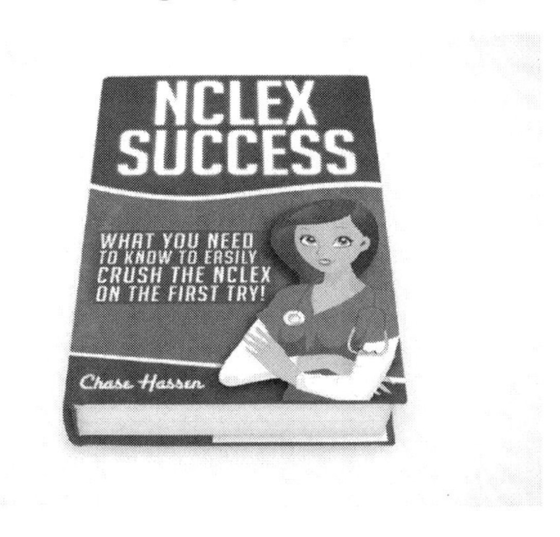

Just to say thanks for downloading my book, I wanted to give you another resource to help you absolutely crush the NCLEX Exam.

For a limited time, you can download this book for FREE.
http://bit.ly/1MPBw86

HIGHLY RECOMMENDED BOOKS
FOR SUCCESS

NCLEX: Cardiovascular System : 105 Nursing Practice and Rationales to Easily Crush the NCLEX!

http://amzn.to/1Rzpn7t

NCLEX: Emergency Nursing: 105 Practice Questions and Rationales to Easily Crush the NCLEX!

http://amzn.to/1RWRLCs

Lab Values: 137 Values You Know to Easily Pass The NCLEX!

http://amzn.to/23afvF9

EKG Interpretation: 24 Hours or Less to Easily Pass the ECG Portion of the NCLEX!

http://amzn.to/1SM1mcw

Fluid and Electrolytes: 24 Hours or Less to Absolutely Crush the NCLEX Exam!

http://amzn.to/1pZd21V

NCLEX: Endocrine System : 105 Nursing Practice Questions and Rationales to EASILY Crush the NCLEX!

http://amzn.to/224ZgXt

NCLEX: Integumentary System : 105 Nursing Practice Questions and Rationales to Easily Crush the NCLEX!

http://amzn.to/23afAJ9

NCLEX: Respiratory System : 105 Nursing Practice Questions and Rationales to Easily Crush the NCLEX!

http://amzn.to/1UPcvgv

INTRODUCTION

This book will teach you the core components of the medical language in 45 minutes or less!

Medical terminology has worked its way into popular culture so that many root forms of medical words are part of everyday life. We do "cardio", which is a root form of medical terms dealing with the heart. In medicine, the root form "cardio" is worked into terms like "cardiology", which means the study of the heart, and "cardiomyopathy", which means a condition of the heart muscle. Once you know the various root forms, most of which are based on Greek or Latin, as well as the prefixes and suffixes that help you narrow down the actual meaning of the word, you will be set to know hundreds of medical words.

It may be helpful for you to create flashcards, which will give you the basic parts of each word. Remember which parts of the word are root words, prefixes and suffixes and then read a medical textbook or article, making the difficult words much simpler when you partition out the parts of the word. In that way, you can identify that the word colonoscopy means colon/oscopy and will know that it means looking at the colon with a lighted camera. There are very few medical terms that aren't set out in just this way. By doing this, you can divide and conquer many different medical words without difficulty. The more you study the cards, the better will your skill be at identifying the various words.

As I explain in the first chapter, medical terminology can appear to be challenging but don't let that scare you. We will discuss what you need to know to gradually take you to more and more advanced words. This book is structured to break down the basic word components that are used to build each medical term. I have a lot to share with you so let's dive in!

CHAPTER 1:
BASIC ELEMENTS OF A MEDICAL WORD

Medical terminology can appear to be a complicated language only understood by members of the medical field but you can certainly learn it, too! As we dive into Chapter 1, I will help you understand that all medical terms are comprised of four basic building blocks that will help you break down and decipher even the most complicated medical terms. After reading and understanding this chapter, you will be able to:

- Define the four basic elements used in building medical terminology.
- Identify which of the four elements are included in each medical term.

1 Basic Word Elements

The first section of this chapter will be spent studying the basic word elements that make up medical terminology. The four basic word elements used in medical terminology are:

- Word Roots
- Combining Forms
- Suffixes

- Prefixes

1.1 Word Roots

The first word element is called a word root. A word root is the portion of the medical term that defines its primary meaning. Every medical term will have at least one word root. Most word roots are derived from either Greek or Latin. Latin roots are primary used to identify parts of the human anatomy and Greek roots are primary used to identify a disease, medical condition, or treatment of the disease or condition. Some examples of word roots are outlined in Table 1-1.

English Term	Word Root
Tissue	hist
Neck or Cervix	cervic
Esophagus	esophag
Blood	hemat

Table 1-1-1: Examples of common English words with their corresponding medical word root

1.2 Combining Forms

A combining form is made when a vowel, known as the combining vowel, is added to a word root. Most combining forms use the letter o, but sometimes the letter I may be used. This vowel allows the joining of two word elements and is the basis for combining the basic elements into complete, complex medical terms. Some examples of combining forms are outlined in Table 1-2.

English Term	Word Root	Combining Form
Tissue	hist	hist/o
Neck	cervic	cervic/o
Esophagus	esophag	esophag/o
Blood	hemat	hemat/o

Table 1-1-2: Examples of common English words with their corresponding medical word root and combining form

1.3 Suffixes

A suffix is the word element added to the end of the term and controls the term's definition. Changing the suffix will change the meaning of the word even when the word root is the same. Some examples of suffixes are outlined in Table 1-3.

Word Root	Combining Form	Suffix	Medical Term
hist	hist/o	-logy	histology
cervic	cervic/o	-itis	cervicitis
esophag	esophage/o	-itis	esophagitis
hemat	hemat/o	-itis	hematitis

Table 1-1-3: Examples of using suffixes with combining forms to derive medical terms

1.4 Prefixes

A prefix is the word element that is added to the beginning of the medical term. Just like the suffix, a prefix controls the term's definition. A good example of this would be the prefixes macro (large) and micro (small). However, a prefix isn't always used. Prefixes are most commonly used to identify a number, position, or negation. Some common prefixes are outlined in Table 1-4

Prefix	Word Root	Suffix	Medical Term
ante-	cubit	-al	antecubital
hypo-	therm	-ia	hyperthermia
medi-	otars	-al	mediotarsal
oxy-	eco	-ia	oxyecoia

Table 1-1-4: Examples of using prefixes with word roots and suffixes to derive medical terms

CHAPTER 2:
RULES TO DEFINING AND BUILDING MEDICAL TERMINOLOGY

Defining medical terms and breaking those terms down to their basic word elements are two vital skills to mastering and understanding medical terminology. Chapter 2 focuses on identifying general guidelines, or rules, that can be used to accomplish these tasks. By reading and understanding this chapter you will be able to:

- Identify the 3 rules to defining medical terminology.
- Identify the 3 rules to building medical terminology.
- Define medical Terminology and separate medical terminology into their basic word elements.

1 The 3 Rules, or Steps, to Defining Medical Terminology

The first step in mastering medical terminology is to be able to define the term. Every medical term can be defined by following these 3 simple steps:

- Identify and define the suffix of the medical term
- Identify and define the first word element of the medical term

- Identify and define the middle word element of the medical term

These examples will help clarify the role of the three rules in defining medical terminology.

Example 1

Use the 3 rules to defining medical terminology to define myocarditis.

Rule 1: Identify and define the suffix of the medical term

Looking at the work myocarditis the suffix is -itis which means inflammation

Rule 2: Identify and define the first word element of the medical term

The first word element in this example is the prefix myo- which means having a relationship to a muscle

Rule 3: Identify and define the middle word element of the medical term

The middle word element in this example is the word root "card" which means "heart".

Putting these together we determine the definition of myocarditis is inflammation of the heart muscle.

Example 2

Use the 3 rules to defining medical terminology to define histology

Rule 1: Identify and define the suffix of the medical term

Looking at the word histology the suffix is -logy which means "study of".

Rule 2: Identify and define the first word element of the medical term

The first word element in this example is the combining form histo- which means tissue.

Rule 3: Identify and define the middle word element of the medical term

In this example, there is no middle word element.

Putting these together we determine the definition of histology is the study of tissue.

2 The 3 Rules, or Steps, to Building Medical Terminology

The second step to mastering medical terminology is to understand how the words are constructed. Any medical term can be built by following these 3 simple rules:

- A word root links a suffix that begins with a vowel
- A combining form links a suffix that begins with a consonant
- A combining form links a root to another root to from a compound word, even when the second root starts with a vowel.

The following examples will help you understand how each rule is used when building medical terminology.

Example 1

Using ***Rule 1***, breakdown gastrectomy into its base word elements.

gastr (word root) + ectomy (suffix) = gastrectomy

Example 2

Using ***Rule 2***, breakdown thoracotomy into its base word elements.

thoraco (combining form) + tomy (suffix) = thoracotomy

Example 3

Using ***Rule 3***, breakdown osteoarthritis into its base word elements.

osteo (combining form) + arthr (word root) + itis (suffix) = osteoarthritis

CHAPTER 3: TYPES OF PREFIXES

As we learned in Chapter 1, prefixes are added to the beginning of a medical term to help control the term's definition. In Chapter 3, we will be learning more about the specific types of prefixes, their use, and how they change the terms definition. After completing and understanding Chapter 3 you will be able to:

- Identify the different types of prefixes and give examples of each
- Identify the prefix in a given medical term and explain how it changes the terms definition
- Understand how prefixes are linked to word roots and combining forms in the creation of medical terminology

1 Prefix Linking

Most medical terms will be made up of one or more word roots or combining forms, and a suffix. Prefixes can be linked to the beginning of the medical term and are used to alter the meaning of the term. For example in the term "peri-" is a prefix meaning "around the time of" and "post-" is a prefix meaning "after the time of". Adding these prefixes to the word "mortal" gives you "perimortal" (around the time of death) and "postmortal" (after the time of death). Table 3-1 has an additional example of how linking different prefixes can change the words meaning.

Prefix	**Word Root**	**Suffix**	**Medical Term**	**Meaning**
hyper	thyroid	ism	hyperthyroidism	condition where the thyroid produces excessive hormones
hypo	thyroid	ism	hypothyroidism	condition where the thyroid under produces hormones

Table 3-1: Example of how changing the prefix alters the meaning of the medical term

2 Types of Prefixes

There are four main types of prefixes. They are:

- Prefixes of position
- Prefixes of number
- Prefixes of measurement
- Prefixes of direction

There are also some other common prefixes that don't fall into one of the four main categories.

2.1 Prefixes of Position

Prefixes of position are used to describe a place or location. The prefixes of position are:

- hypo
- infra
- sub
- inter
- post
- pre
- pro
- retro
- epi

2.2 Using prefixes of position

The following sentences illustrate the use of prefixes of position. The medical term containing the prefix is underlined.

Some people get epigastric pain if they lie down too quickly after eating.

Word analysis:

epi above

gastr stomach

ic pertaining to

pertaining to above the stomach

Diabetics use hypodermic needles to inject their insulin.

Word analysis:

hypo under

derm skin

ic pertaining to

pertaining to under the skin

The diaphragm is part of the infracostal anatomy.

Word analysis:

infra below

cost ribs

al pertaining to

pertaining to below the ribs

A subnasal lip lift is one example of a procedure performed by a plastic surgeon.

Word analysis:

sub below

nas nose

al pertaining to

pertaining to below the nose

Studies have shown that using interdental brushes will reduce your risk of gum disease.

Word analysis:

inter between

dent teeth

al pertaining to

pertaining to between the teeth

Most deaths in newborns occur during the postnatal period.

Word analysis:

post after

nat birth

al pertaining to

pertaining to after birth.

Lamaze is one example of a prenatal class.

Word analysis:

pre before

nat birth

al pertaining to

pertaining to before birth

Prognosis is defined as a prediction of the course and end of a disease and the estimated chance of recovery.

Word analysis:

pro before

gnosis knowing

knowing before

Retroversion of the uterus refers to tipping backward of

the uterus from its normal position.

Word analysis:

Retro backward

version turning

turning backward

2.3 Prefixes of number

Prefixes of number are used to describe quantities. The prefixes of number are:

- bi
- dipl
- diplo
- hemi
- mono
- uni
- multi
- poly
- primi
- quadri
- tri

2.4 Using prefixes of number

The following sentences illustrate the use of prefixes of number. The medical term containing the prefix is underlined.

The patient suffered from a <u>bilateral</u> pleural effusion.

Word analysis:

bi two

later sides

al pertaining to

pertaining to two sides

The patient's diplopia makes it hard for her to walk.

Word analysis:

dipl double

opia vision

Double vision

Diplobacterial reproduction is seen in bacteria that are joined in pairs.

Word analysis:

diplo double

Bacerti bacteria

al pertaining to

pertaining to double bacteria – bacteria that links in pairs

The accident caused the patient to suffer from hemiplegia.

Word analysis:

hemi half

plegia paralysis

half paralysis or paralysis of half of the body

Infections are commonly treated using a monotherapy consisting of an antibiotic.

Word analysis:

mono one

therapy treatment

One treatment; a treatment involving a single medication

Cell fusion is the process where two or more uninuclear cells join to become a multinuclear cell.

Word analysis:

uni one

nucle nucleus

ar pertaining to

pertaining to one nucleus

multi more than one

nucle nucleus

ar pertaining to

pertaining to more than one nucleus

People who are scared of more than one thing suffer from polyphobia.

Word analysis:

poly many

phobia fear

many fears or fear of many things

Women who become pregnant for the first time are medically known as primigravida.

Word analysis:

prima first

gravida pregnant woman

First pregnant woman or woman in her first pregnancy

Quadriplegia is an extreme example of a consequence from a car accident.

Word analysis:

quadri four

plegia paralysis

paralysis of four limbs

Triceps describes a muscle arising by three heads with a single insertion. One example of this would be the triceps brachii of the posterior arm.

Word analysis:

tri three

ceps head

Three heads

2.5 Prefixes of measurement

Prefixes of measurement show a quantity or degree of involvement. The prefixes of measurement are:

- hyper
- macro
- micro

2.6 Using prefixes of measurement

The following sentences illustrate the use of prefixes of measurement. The medical term containing the prefix is underlined.

The patient`s blood work showed that he was suffering from hypercalcemia.

Word analysis:

hyper	excessive
calc	calcium
emia	blood condition

Excessive calcium blood condition or excessive calcium in the blood

A macroglobulin is defined as a plasma globulin with a high molecular weight.

Word analysis:

macro	large

globulin protein

large protein

Microscopes are used to see things that are too small to see with the naked eye.

Word analysis:

micro small

scope instrument for examining

small instrument for examining or instrument for examining small things

2.7 Prefixes of direction

Prefixes of direction are used to indicate a pathway or route. The prefixes of direction are:

- ab
- ad
- circum
- peri
- dia
- trans
- ecto
- eso
- exo
- extra
- endo
- intra
- para
- super
- supra
- ultra

2.8 Using prefixes of direction

The following sentences illustrate the use of prefixes of direction. The medical term containing the prefix is underlined.

Kicking your leg sideways is an example of abduction.

Word analysis:

ab	from or away from
duction	act of leading or bringing

leading away from; movement of a limb away from the body

Covering your mouth when you sneeze is an example of an adduction.

Word analysis:

ad	toward
duction	act of leading or bringing

bringing toward; movement of a limb towards the body

There are many blood vessels that are circumrenal.

Word analysis:

circum	around
ren	kidney
al	pertaining to

pertaining to around the kidney

Labor is one activity that will occur in the perinatal period.

Word analysis:

peri around

nat birth

al pertaining to

pertaining to around birth

It is challenging working when you have diarrhea.

Word analysis:

dia through, across

rrhea discharge or flow

flow through

A transvaginal ultrasound is often used in getting a clearer picture of a women`s reproductive organs than a normal ultrasound will give.

Word analysis:

trans through, across

vagin vagina

al pertaining to

pertaining to across or through the vagina

An ectogenous liver cyst forms outside of the liver.

Word analysis:

ecto outside, outward

gen forming, producing, origin

ous pertaining to

pertaining to forming outside the body or structure

Esotropia and Exotropia are two eye conditions that can be found in newborns.

Word analysis:

eso inward

exo outward

tropia turning

inward or outward turning of the eyes

Scientists are studying the effect of extracranial injuries on the outcome of traumatic brain injury patients.

Word analysis:

extra outside

crani cranium or skull

al pertaining to

pertaining to outside of the cranium or skull

The endocrine system consists of glands that secrete hormones directly into the blood stream.

Word analysis:

endo in, within

crine	secrete

secrete within

Vitamin B12 shots are often given through intramuscular injections.

Word analysis:

intra	in, within
muscul	muscle
ar	pertaining to

pertaining to within the muscle

The parathyroid glands are adjacent to the thyroid.

Word analysis:

para	near, beside, beyond
thyroid	thyroid

near or beside the thyroid

The superior vena cava carries deoxygenated blood from the upper half of the body to the heart.

Word analysis:

super	upper
ior	pertaining to

pertaining to the upper part of a structure

An ultrasound uses ultrasonic waves to produce images of body parts that can then be used to diagnose patients.

Word analysis:

ultra	excess, beyond
son	sound
ic	pertaining to

pertaining to sound beyond; often sound beyond human hearing.

2.9 Other common prefixes

There are a number of common prefixes that don`t fit into one of the four main categories. They are:

- a
- an
- anti
- contra
- brady
- dys
- eu
- hetero
- homo
- homeo
- mal
- pan
- pseudo
- syn
- tachy

2.10 Using the other common prefixes

The following sentences illustrate the use of the other common prefixes. The medical term containing the prefix is underlined.

Some breast cancer survivors may suffer from amastia.

Word analysis:

a	without, not
mast	breast
ia	condition

a condition without breasts

Patients who undergo surgery will often be given anesthesia.

Word analysis:

an	without
esthesia	feeling

without feeling

Washing your hands with an antibacterial soap can help prevent the spread of germs.

Word analysis:

anti	against
bacteri	bacteria
al	pertaining to

pertaining to against bacteria

Condoms are one popular method of contraception.

Word analysis:

contra	against

ception conceiving

against conception

Bradycardia can be a life threatening condition.

Word analysis:

brady slow

cardia heart

slow heart or slow heart rate

Some women are more prone to dystocia than others.

Word analysis:

dys bad, painful, or difficult

tocia childbirth, labor

difficult labor

CHAPTER 4:
TYPES OF SUFFIXES

As we learned in Chapter 1, suffixes are added to the end of a medical term to help control the term's definition. In Chapter 4, we will be learning more about the specific types of suffixes, their use, and how they change the term's definition. After completing and understanding Chapter 4 you will be able to:

- Identify the different types of suffixes and give examples of each
- Identify the suffix in a given medical term and explain how it changes the term's definition
- Understand how suffixes are linked to word roots and combining forms in the creation of medical terminology

1 Suffix Linking

Suffixes are linked to the end of the medical term and are used to alter the meaning of the term. For example -itis is a suffix meaning inflammation and logy is a suffix meaning the study of. Adding these suffixes to the word root hemat gives you hematitis (inflammation of the blood vessels) and hematology (the study of blood). Table 4-1 has an additional example of how linking different suffixes can change the words meaning.

Word Root	Suffix	Medical Term	Meaning
colon/o	scope	colonoscope	Thin flexible tube used to look at the colon
colon/o	scopy	colonoscopy	Diagnostic test that allows visual inspection of the colon

Table 4-1: Example of how changing the suffix changes the meaning of the medical term

You will also recall from chapter one that suffix linking follows 3 basic rules:

- A word root links a suffix that begins with a vowel
- A combining form links a suffix that begins with a consonant
- A combining form links a root to another root to from a compound word, even when the second root starts with a vowel.

2 Three Main Categories of Suffixes

Grouping suffixes by category makes it easier to remember them, and is an effective way to learn medical terminology. The three main categories of suffixes are:

- Surgical
- Diagnostic, Pathological, and Related
- Grammatical

2.1 Surgical Suffixes

Surgical suffixes are used to describe invasive surgical procedures. The surgical suffixes are:

- centesis
- clasis
- desis
- ectomy
- lysis
- pexy
- plasty
- rrhaphy
- stomy
- tome
- tomy
- tripsy

2.2 Using Surgical Suffixes

The following sentences will illustrate the use of some of the surgical suffixes. The word with the suffix will be underlined.

After getting into an accident, it was determined that John would need a <u>cardiocentesis</u> to drain the blood around his heart.

Word analysis:

cardio heart

centesis surgical puncture

surgical puncture of the heart

An <u>osteoclasis</u> may be required in a broken bone isn't set properly to ensure complete recovery.

Word analysis

oste/o bone

clasis to break; surgical fracture

surgically break bone often to repair a deformity

After suffering from tonsillitis most of his life, John finally went to the hospital for a <u>tonsillectomy</u>.

Word analysis:

tonsil tonsils

ectomy excision, removal

removal of the tonsils

To help her feel younger, Eleanor elected to see a plastic surgeon for a <u>mastopexy</u>.

Word analysis:

mast/o breast

pexy fixation

fixation of the breast(s)

An <u>osteotome</u> is a surgical chisel used to cut through bone

Word analysis

oste/o bone

tome surgical instrument to cut

surgical instrument to cut bone

After regular intubation failed, doctors performed a tracheotomy to help the patient breathe.

Word analysis:

trache/o trachea

tomy incision

incision into the trachea

2.3 Diagnostic, Pathological, and Related Suffixes

Diagnostic suffixes describe a procedure or test used to identify an illness, or the tool used to perform the test. Pathological suffixes describe the illness itself. The diagnostic, pathological, and related suffixes are:

- Diagnostic
- gram
- graph
- graphy
- meter
- metry
- scope
- scopy
- Pathological and Related
- algia
- dynia
- cele
- ectasis
- edema
- emesis
- emia
- gen
- genesis
- iasis
- itis
- lith
- malacia
- megaly
- oma
- osis
- pathy
- penia

- phagia
- phasia
- phobia
- plasia
- plasm
- plegia
- ptosis
- rrhage
- rrhagia
- rrhea
- rrhexis
- sclerosis
- spasm
- stenosis
- toxic
- trophy

2.4 Using Diagnostic, Pathological, and Related Suffixes

Yearly physicals often include an electrocardiogram to check for heart defects.

Word analysis:

electr/o	electricity
cardi/o	heart
gram	record, writing

record of electrical activity of the heart

After suffering from a heart attack, Steve was sent for an angiography.

Word analysis:

angi/o	vessel
graphy	process of recording

process of recording blood vessels

Doctors use colonoscopes to visually inspect the colon of patients. This process is known as a colonoscopy.

Word analysis:

colon/o colon

scope instrument for examining

instrument for examining a colon

colon/o colon

scopy visual examination

visual examination of the colon

The medical term for an earache is otodynia.

Word analysis:

ot/o ear

dynia pain

pain in the ear

A common cause of lymphedema is a blockage in the lymph vessels.

Word analysis:

lymph lymph

edema swelling

swelling and accumulation of lymph fluid

Severe flu systems may include hyperemesis.

Word analysis:

hyper	excessive
emesis	vomiting

excessive vomiting

Asbestos was a common insulation until it was discovered to be a carcinogen.

Word analysis:

carcin/o	cancer
gen	forming, producing, origin

producing cancer

Severe cholelithiasis often will require a cholecystectomy.

Word analysis:

chol/e	bile, gall
lith	stone, calculus
iasis	abnormal condition

abnormal condition of gallstones.

Arthritis is a painful condition that affects mostly elderly people.

Word analysis:

arthr joints

itis inflammation

joint inflammation

Cardiomegaly refers to an abnormal enlargement of the heart.

Word analysis:

cardi/o heart

megaly enlargement

enlargement of the heart

The medical term for decrease of red blood cells is erythropenia.

Word analysis:

erythr/o red

penia decrease, deficiency

decrease in red blood cells

Extreme sore throats might cause temporary dysphagia.

Word analysis:

dys bad, painful, or difficult

phagia eating, swallowing

inability or difficulty in swallowing

One common side effect of a stroke is aphasia.

Word analysis:

a without, not

phasia speech

absence or impairment of speech

An arteriorrhexis is one of the main causes of a Hemorrhage.

Word analysis:

hem/o blood

rrhage bursting forth (of)

bursting forth of blood

arteri/o artery

rrhexis rupture

rupture of an artery

Chronic arteriostenosis can lead to high blood pressure, heart attacks, and even death.

Word analysis:

arteri/o artery

stenosis hardening

abnormal hardening of an artery

Mercury is an example of a neurotoxic substance.

Word analysis:

neur/o nerve

toxic poison

poisonous to nerves

2.5 Grammatical Suffixes

Grammatical suffixes are attached to word roots to form adjectives, nouns, and singular or plural forms of medical terminology. Grammatical suffixes c an also be used to from diminutive forms of medical terminology. The grammatical suffixes are:

- Adjectives
- ac
- al
- ar
- ary
- eal
- ic
- ical
- ile
- ior
- ous
- tic

- Nouns
- esis
- ia
- ism
- iatry
- ician
- ist
- y
- Diminutive
- icle
- ole
- ule

2.6 Using Grammatical Suffixes

The following sentences are illustrations of using grammatical suffixes. The word with the suffix will be underlined.

Pneumonia is a common pulmonary disease.

Word analysis:

Pulmon lung

ary pertaining to

pertaining to the lungs

pneumon air, lung

ia condition

lung condition; usually an infection caused by bacteria, viruses, or disease

The circulatory system is comprised of arteries, arterioles, and capillaries.

Word analysis:

ateri artery

ole small, minute

small artery

CONCLUSION

I hope this book was helpful for you to learn the fundamentals of Medical Terminology!

Now you know the various root words and their meanings. Some words will have similar meanings but don't let that get you down. If they have similar meanings, the suffix will usually tease out the actual meaning of the word. Suffixes can be the most difficult thing to learn because they are almost all short nonsensical syllables that have a wide array of meanings. They basically have to be memorized so that you can better define the meaning of the word.

Final Quiz

Here are some medical terms. Find the prefixes, root words, and suffixes so that you can better define the word. Good luck!

Questions

1. Pericarditis
2. Schistosomiasis
3. Prenatal

4. Jejunostomy
5. Pericardiocentesis
6. Craniotomy
7. Angiography
8. Hysteroscopy
9. Hysterectomy
10. Pleurodynia

Answers

1. Peri/card/itis which means "inflammation around the heart"
2. Schistosom'iasis which means " a disease of having Schistosoma parasite"
3. Pre/natal which means "before birth"
4. Jejuno/stomy which means "a hole or opening in the jejunum"
5. Peri/cardio/centesis which means "puncturing a hole around the heart"
6. Crani/otomy which means "an opening to the brain or skull"
7. Angio/graphy which means " a measurement of the blood vessels"
8. Hystero/scopy which means "using a scope to see the uterus"
9. Hyster/ectomy which means "removal of the uterus"
10. Pleuro/dyn/ia which means "a condition of pain in the lungs"

Made in the USA
Lexington, KY
26 February 2019